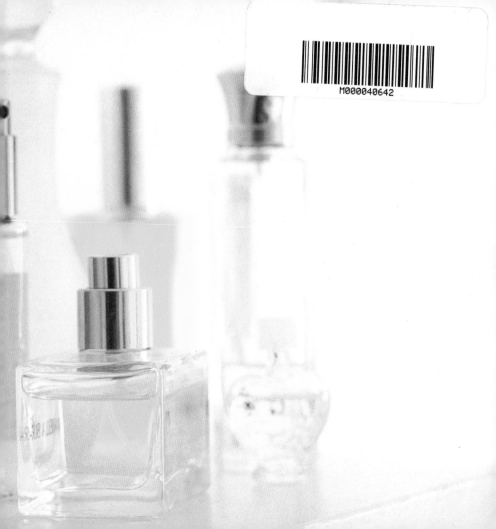

M000040642

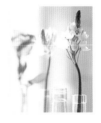

refreshing

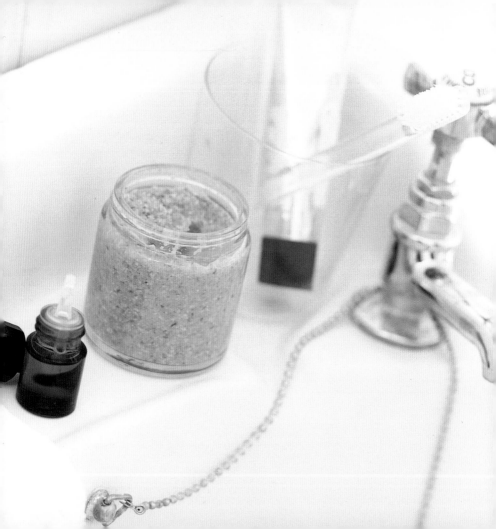

home spa

refreshing

Liz Wilde

RYLAND
PETERS
& SMALL

LONDON NEW YORK

Senior Designer Megan Smith
Senior Editor Clare Double
Picture Researcher Tracy Ogino
Production Paul Harding
Art Director Anne-Marie Bulat
Editorial Director Julia Charles
Publishing Director Alison Starling

First published in the United States in 2006
by Ryland Peters & Small
519 Broadway, 5th Floor
New York, NY 10012
www.rylandpeters.com

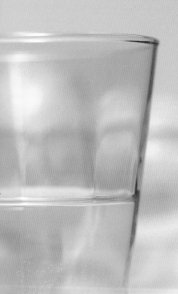

If you are in any doubt about your health, please
consult your doctor before making any changes to
your usual dietary and wellbeing regime. Essential
oils are very powerful and potentially toxic if used
too liberally. Please follow the guidelines and never
use the oils neat on bare skin, unless advised
otherwise. This book is not suitable for anyone
during pregnancy.

contents

introduction

How can you give the best of yourself to your work, family, and friends when you're running on empty?

Taking care of yourself not only makes you look lighter and brighter (think clear skin, glossy hair, and a better body), it also makes you feel so much better, with balanced moods, deeper sleep, and significantly reduced stress levels.

A 21st-century lifestyle means you may be neglecting important parts of your body and mind. You weren't meant to spend the majority of your time indoors, sitting in front of a computer or a TV set. Your body wasn't designed to eat processed food and take little exercise. Add to that a sight and sound overload (how many emails did you read today? how many opinions have you heard?), while your senses of smell and touch, which are linked to your emotions, are deprived.

We can get sick if our immune system is weak, and regular amounts of stress (doing too much, no time to relax, putting yourself last) will decrease your body's ability to fight disease. More than 80% of visits to the doctor are stress-related, and scientists now know that

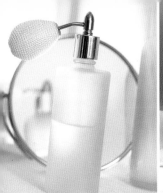
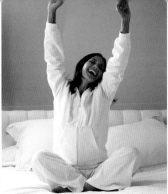
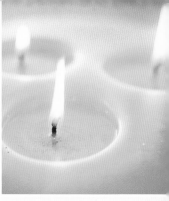

there's a link between emotions and your immune system, which proves how much of your health is in your own hands.

This means that spending time looking after yourself and satisfying your forgotten senses is good for your health. So what are you waiting for? Lock the bathroom door and indulge in some nurturing rituals.

You're probably reading this because you feel run-down and tired, but if you regularly use the techniques in this book you'll be well on your way to a happier, healthier life. Aim to save at least 20 minutes a day to spoil yourself, and help your body heal from the inside with a less toxic lifestyle, regular exercise, and good nutrition. Learn to look after yourself and you'll be able to do everything else so much better.

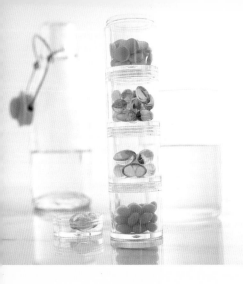

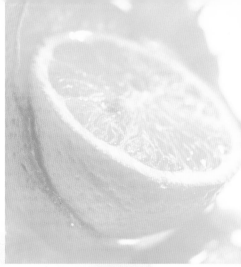

Wellbeing is attained little by little, and is no little thing itself.
Zeno of Citium

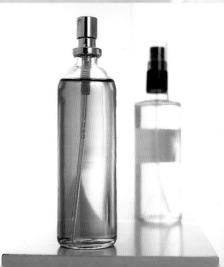

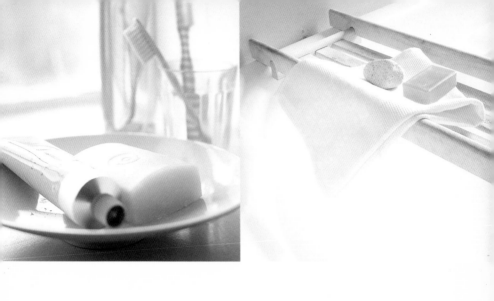

rescue

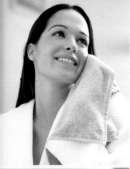

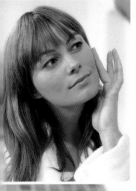

botox-free skin boosters

Everyone has days when they wake up feeling pale and blotchy. Instead of hiding away, throw open the window (no matter what the weather) and take some slow, deep breaths.

Even better, go for a walk, dance around to your favorite CD, or do some yoga. Next, remove your cleanser using a lintfree cloth wrung out in warm water, then soak it in cold and lie the cloth over your face for a few seconds to **CALM ANY REDNESS**. Apply your moisturizer by dotting it on lightly with the pads of your fingers (the right moisturizer will make your skin look and feel more springy for up to six hours afterwards), and then eat breakfast before putting on your makeup, to give it time to sink in.

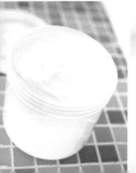

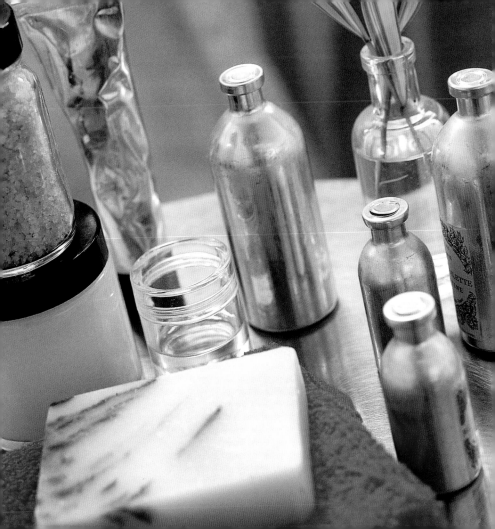

hair S.O.S.

According to trichologist Philip Kingsley, drinking a moderate amount of alcohol can actually be good for your hair (what a great excuse!). It's the smoky, polluted party atmosphere that will leave you smelly and bedraggled.

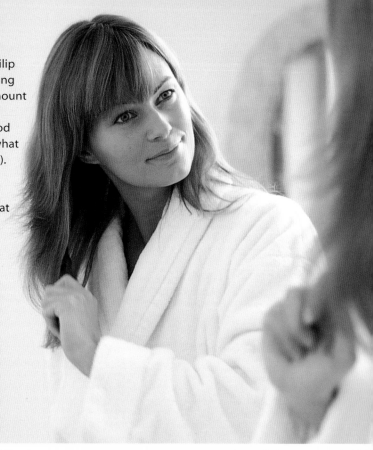

To help your hair's recovery, massage a mixture of witch hazel and vodka (equal measures) into your scalp for a few minutes, then rinse and shampoo as normal. To **GIVE YOUR HAIR A BOOST** before a big night, shake together two tablespoons each of witch hazel, vodka, and mouthwash, and knead into your scalp for five minutes. Apply a rich conditioner over the top, cover your head in a shower cap, and leave on for 15 minutes. And be warned: **INSUFFICIENT RINSING** is the most common cause of dull hair and itchy scalps, so if you usually dunk in sudsy bath water, finish with a rinse under the shower.

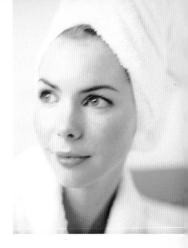

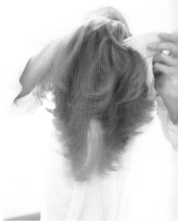

morning-after makeup

Looking less than your best? Makeup was created for off days, but resist the temptation to trowel it on, as you'll make dehydrated skin look worse.

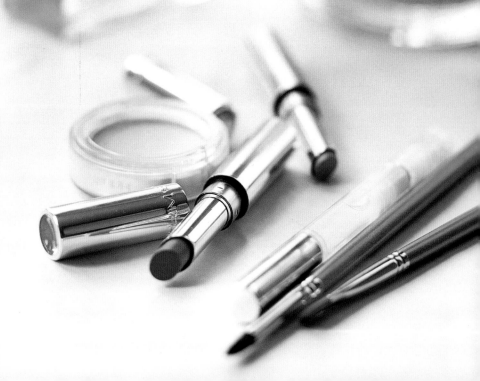

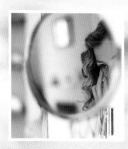

Begin by moisturizing twice (leave 5–10 minutes between applications to give the cream time to sink in), then apply a **SKIN BRIGHTENER** to do just that. Foundation should be kept to a minimum (apply with a stubby brush just where you need to cover morning-after blotches), and skip powder unless you're very shiny. Brown or gray mascara is far softer than black is on red, puffy eyes, and a cream blusher is more flattering than powder (choose tawny-based shades rather than pink, which will only emphasize high coloring). And apply a slightly brighter lipstick than usual to add color to your face. Just keep it **SHEER AND GLOSSY**, so the effect is more sophisticated than startling.

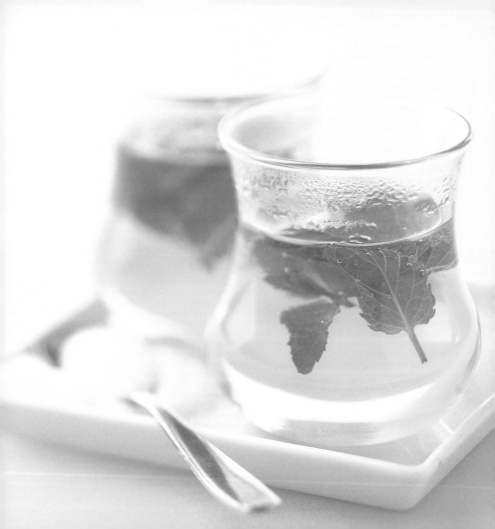

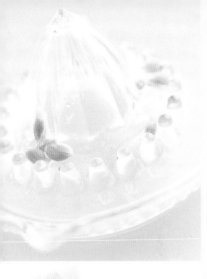

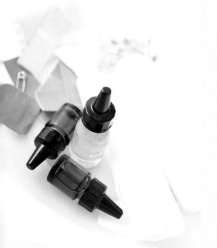

natural remedies for off days

- **BLOATING** Drink a glass of hot water with a squeeze of lemon.

- **COLD SORE** Apply a few drops of lemon juice or melissa essential oil three times a day.

- **COUGH** Drink a glass of water with fresh honey and lemon.

- **HEADACHE** Dot neat lavender oil onto each temple.

- **NAUSEA** Drink plenty of fennel or peppermint tea.

- **PIMPLES AND GRAZES** Apply neat tea tree oil with a Q-tip three times a day (this also works well on athlete's foot).

look after your liver

Reverse the effects of too much rich food and alcohol by drinking a glass of hot water first thing in the morning and last thing at night, as this gets your bowels moving properly again to clean out all the mucus in your body. The second-best thing you can do for your liver is stick with simple meals including lots of fresh fruit and vegetables (broccoli, cabbage, and cauliflower are extra-efficient at detoxing the liver). This is also the time to get inventive with your blender, as homemade juices head straight for your bloodstream to work a minor miracle. The most effective cleansers are apple, grapefruit, pear, carrot, beet, and watercress.

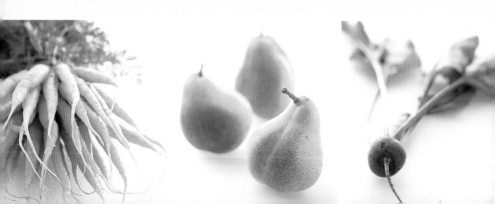

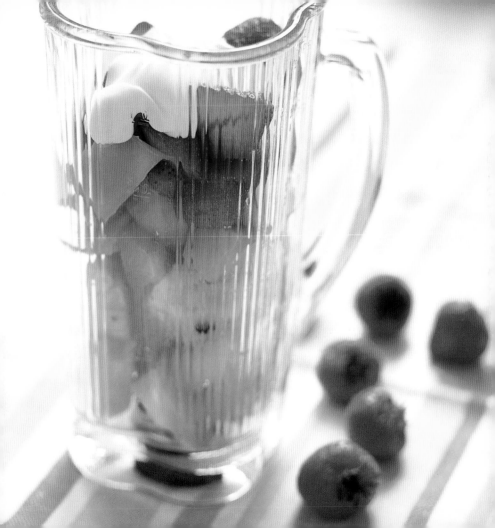

day to night repair work

Repair your day face for nighttime by first spritzing it with water (this makes old makeup easier to blend and also softens fine lines). Then get to work with a light-reflecting concealer to minimize the bad and highlight the good. Apply along the lines that run from nose to mouth and blend with your finger. For under-eye circles, hold your mirror at eye level and, looking ahead, tilt your chin down so you can see exactly where the dark area is. Apply just one line directly underneath (any more will highlight them), then blend well. Places to emphasize include the inside of your eyes next to the tear ducts, your brows, and just above the Cupid's bow of your lips. Don't be tempted to reapply foundation and powder, as it will look cakey. Just use a cover stick to hide any blemishes that have worked their way through during the day. A touch of shimmer shadow directly above your pupils and blended over lids will wake up tired eyes, as will curling your lashes and one more coat of mascara.

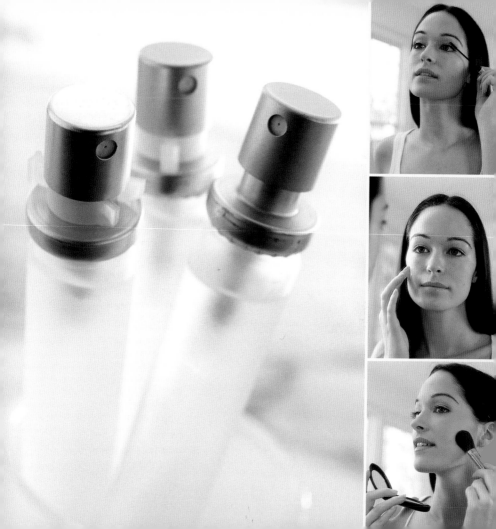

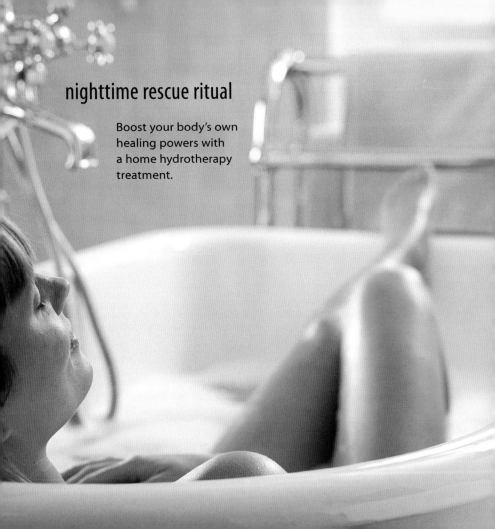

nighttime rescue ritual

Boost your body's own
healing powers with
a home hydrotherapy
treatment.

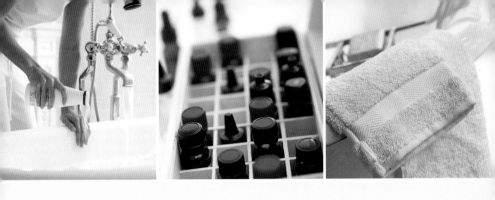

Fill a tub with warm water (90–95°F) and immerse your whole body for a **MILD DETOX** as you sweat (great for minor colds). Stay in for 20 minutes and then jump into a warm bed to prolong the detox effect. Make the experience more pleasurable by adding a combination of aromatherapy oils (5–10 drops in total) to the water, or treat dry skin conditions with 1–2 cups of finely ground oatmeal or a 1-pound box of baking soda. Drink plenty of water afterwards to counteract dehydration.

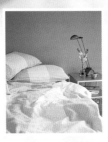

recovery remedies for off days

1 The quickest way to heal is to rest a lot and eat little, so
   your body can concentrate on fighting the enemy. If you
   feel hungry, don't be tempted by comfort food, as even
   a small amount of sugar can reduce your immunity by
   up to half. Fill up on immunity-boosting fruit and
   vegetables instead.

2 Color-corrective fluid or powder can do wonders
   for tired, sallow skin. Choose a lilac shade and apply
   sparingly for luminous skin even under harsh lighting.

3 Do you know what helps you relax? List everything from
   the big and expensive (a weekend away, a massage)
   to the small and free (a home facial, a cuddle). Then
   put the list where you can see it and find time for each
   and every one.

4   A good concealer can hide just about anything, but get the color right or it will sit on the surface of your skin emphasizing exactly what you're trying to hide. The most common mistake is using one that's too pale (a shade lighter than your foundation is as far as you need to go) or too pink (yellow-based shades give the most believable coverage).

5   Blusher is the quickest way to wake up a tired face and works wonders as a mid-afternoon boost. Choose a tawny-pink tone (the most anti-aging) and use a large brush to apply over the apples of your cheeks, chin, and eyelids.

6   Make your eyes look brighter and more awake by feeling for the pressure point on the bridge of your nose (a small dent) and pressing for a count of three.

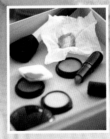

energize

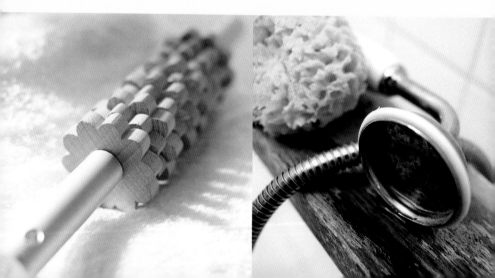

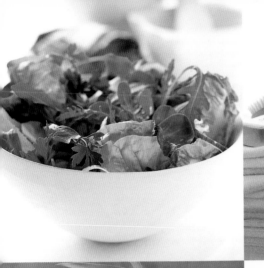

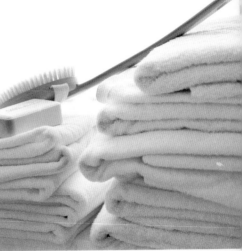

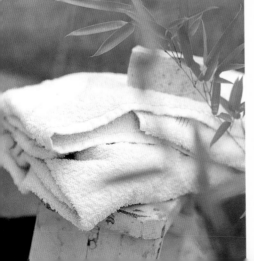

Energy is
eternal delight.
William Blake

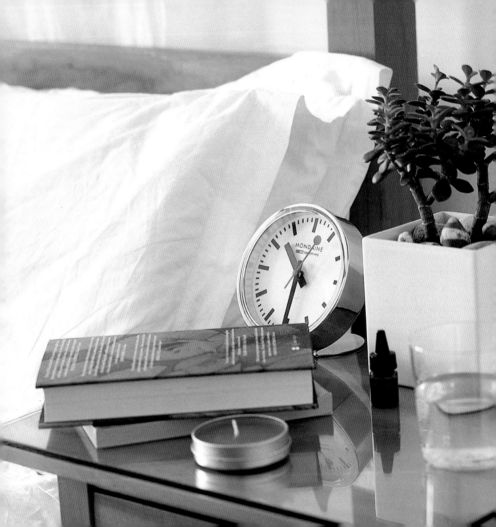

reset your clock

Start your day on a high with this simple wake-up strategy. Before you get out of bed, ask yourself: What is my one exciting thing for today? That way you'll know there's at least one reason to rise and shine. Never enough time in the day? Then turn yourself into a morning person and fill those extra hours with self-care. Set your alarm for 7 A.M. (or before), and get out of bed however tired you feel. By the evening you'll be ready for bed earlier than usual, which will begin to reset your biological clock. Alternatively, do it gradually by setting your alarm 15 minutes earlier every 3–4 days.

graze through your day

Think of eating natural foods as filling your body with premium gasoline. Thousands of years ago we ate small meals every few hours made up of food that was available close by. This gave us energy for hunting and gathering, and if you want to fight fatigue, the same eating habits will work today. Now called grazing, small regular meals of natural plant-based food will give you a smooth, long-lasting high that coffee never can. For instant energizing effects, take a tip from high-school soccer players and copy their half-time habit of sucking on an orange. Need a one-hit wonder? Avocado contains more energy and nutrients than any other fruit.

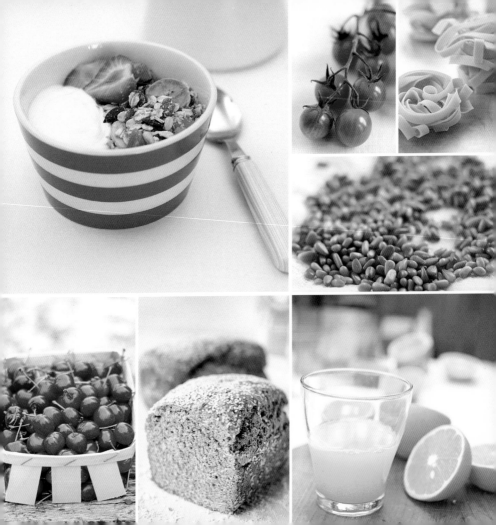

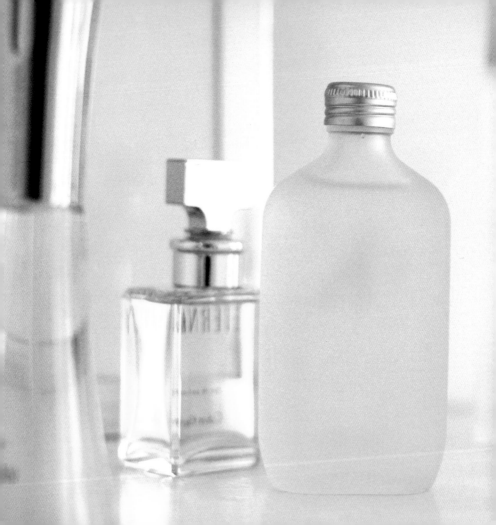

stimulating scents

Don't underestimate the energizing effect of a feel-good fragrance (research shows that 25% of people who lose their sense of smell also lose their sex drive!). Traditionally, scent was applied to neck and wrists, as pulse points 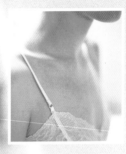 are warm, so they diffuse the smell more quickly. For lasting results apply less, but to more places, such as cleavage, backs of knees, and insides of elbows. And don't forget to scent your surroundings with essential oils for a mid-afternoon boost, or simply sniff the bottle. Energizing oils include bergamot, peppermint, rosemary, lemon, and eucalyptus.

wake up your face

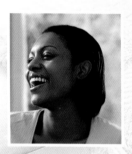

Try these facial yoga moves to wake up your face and release tension. (They tone muscles to prevent sagging, too.)

1 Raise your eyebrows, hold, and repeat three times.

2 Stick out your jaw, hold, and repeat three times. Then clench your back teeth hard, release, and let your jaw drop open. Repeat five times.

3 Puff your cheeks out and hold for three seconds. Then alternate by pushing air into each cheek three times.

4 Suck in your cheeks, hold, and relax.

5 Massage your gums by moving your tongue all around your mouth.

6 Drop your head back and then open and close your mouth five times, feeling the stretch in your neck.

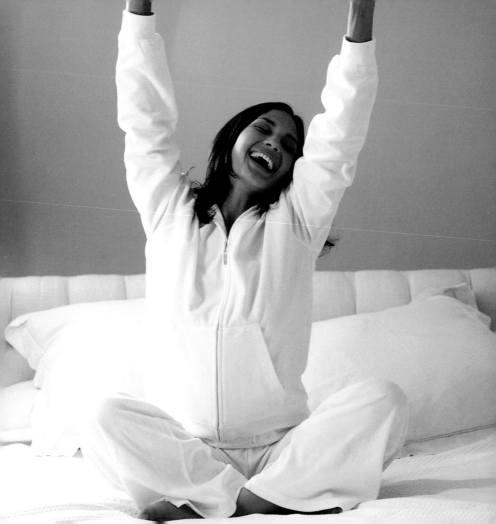

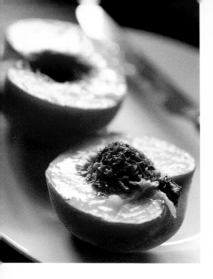

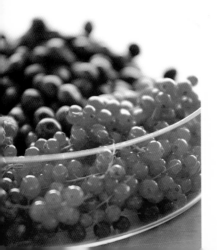

beat your cravings

Food intolerances sap your energy, but, rather than pay for expensive food allergy tests, just look at what you crave. Chances are the very thing you can't imagine living without could be just what you need to give up. The trick is to reduce your intake gradually rather than going cold turkey and forcing your body into shock (think headaches, pimples, or bloating). Simply cut your intake in half in the first week and then cut it in half again in the second. Unless you were feeding your habit continuously, this should get you to a much more manageable level.

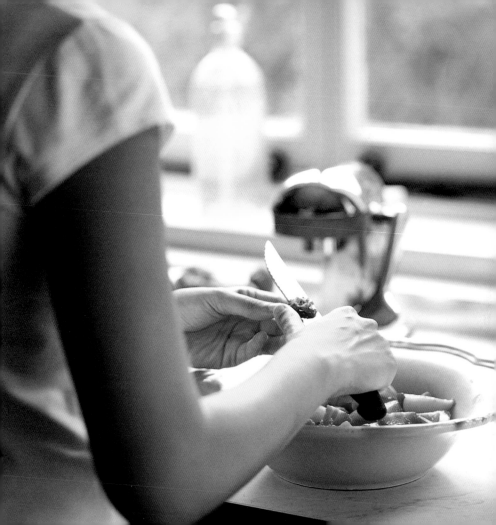

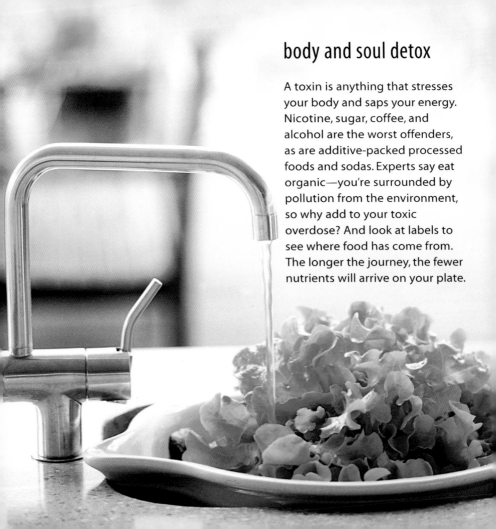

body and soul detox

A toxin is anything that stresses your body and saps your energy. Nicotine, sugar, coffee, and alcohol are the worst offenders, as are additive-packed processed foods and sodas. Experts say eat organic—you're surrounded by pollution from the environment, so why add to your toxic overdose? And look at labels to see where food has come from. The longer the journey, the fewer nutrients will arrive on your plate.

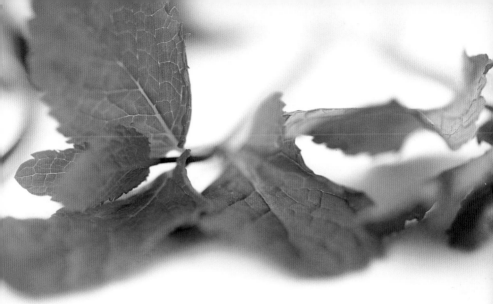

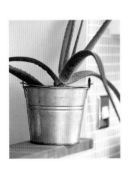

Don't ignore **MIND TOXINS**, either. A stressful job or bad relationship overworks your adrenal glands, playing havoc with your digestion. Reverse the damage by starting your day with a small glass of aloe vera juice. Long known as one of the most beneficial plants on earth, aloe vera enhances energy levels by promoting better absorption of nutrients and helping your body detox naturally.

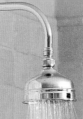

fast energy fixes

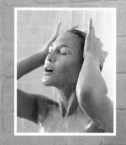

1 Your lymphatic system works like a drain, taking away all the toxins from your body, but it has no pump of its own, so you need to help get things moving. Exercise and massage will do it, but for the quickest fix, turn your shower to cold and stand under it for 10 seconds before turning the water back to warm. Repeat as many times as you can stand.

2 On your commute home, don't read or listen to music. Just be. Doing nothing is wonderfully energizing, as it gives your brain space to slow down and process the day. You don't even need to find a solution to a problem. Just let thoughts pop in and out of your head, and when your brain's ready, it will find the answer—the reason some of your best ideas occur in the bath!

3   It takes extra energy to hold muscles tight, so do your body a favor by taking regular stretch breaks throughout the day.

4   Breathing deeply expels 70% of the toxins in your body. Take a breath in that feels like it's filling up your whole body right from your toes. Hold for a second and then let it all out (gently) through your nose. Or have a yawn—it's your body's natural way of getting more oxygen to your brain.

5   Arousal is a great energizer as it heightens all your senses, making it similar to the energy you'd feel before running a race. Flirting gives you a mini-charge, too, or get your kicks by connecting with high-energy memories. Remember when you fell in love or landed your best-ever job? Relive it in your mind and those endorphins won't be far behind.

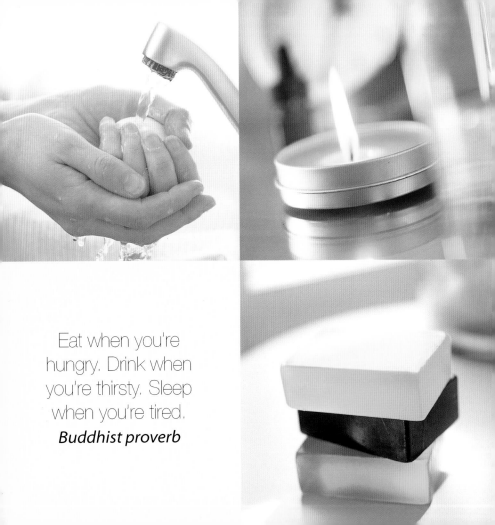

Eat when you're hungry. Drink when you're thirsty. Sleep when you're tired. *Buddhist proverb*

restore

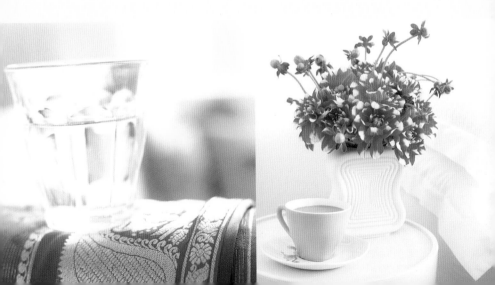

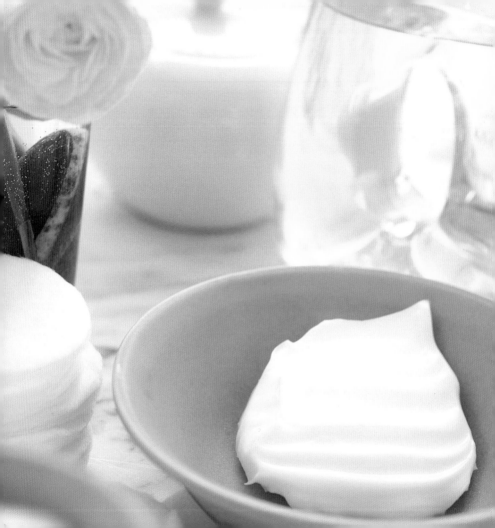

stressed skin solutions

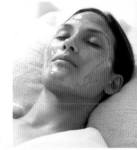

- If your skin regularly looks tired, invest in an **"EMERGENCY" MASK** to instantly revive you. These products contain a cooling, skin-tightening ingredient such as menthol or camphor, and work by boosting the circulation (the reason for that tingle), which stimulates the blood capillaries and gives you a healthy glow.

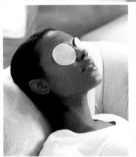

- Give yourself a **QUICK FACELIFT** in the shower by pointing the shower head (don't have the water pressure on too high) at your face for a few minutes. With the water on cool, close your eyes and work in large circles one way and then the other.

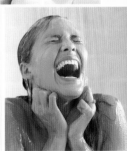

wonderful water

We lose two quarts of water from our bodies every day (before even doing anything strenuous), and without enough water, nothing functions as well as it should.

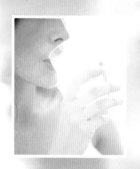

If you suffer mood swings, headaches, fatigue, or even allergic reactions, drinking a minimum of **EIGHT CUPS A DAY** (about two liters, but aim for three) will lessen your symptoms. Monitor your intake by filling a two-liter bottle at the start of the day and congratulating yourself if you need a refill. And drink regularly rather than downing too much in one go, as more than a liter in an hour can upset your body's natural balance.

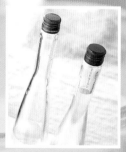

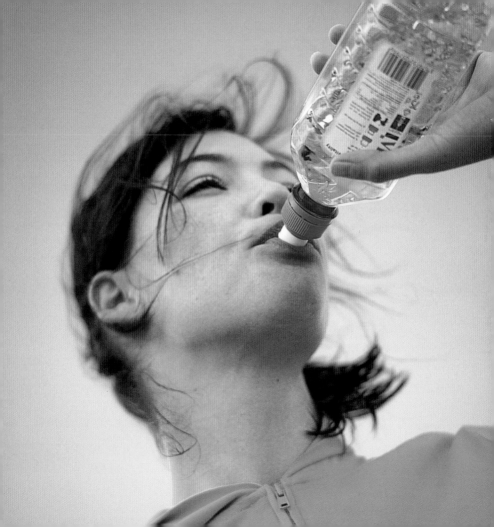

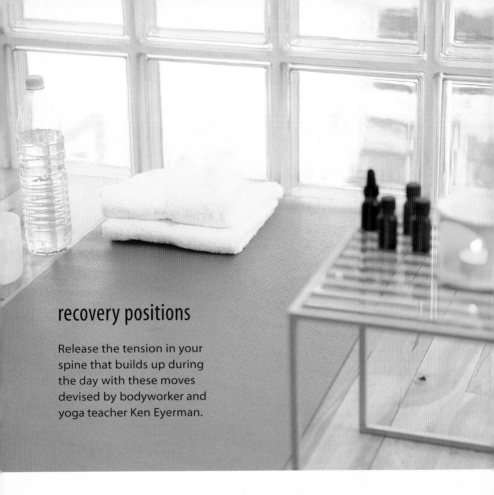

recovery positions

Release the tension in your spine that builds up during the day with these moves devised by bodyworker and yoga teacher Ken Eyerman.

1 Lie flat on the floor with your legs a little way apart. Place one hand on your abdomen and one on your chest so you can feel your breath moving between the two. Then use your fingers to gently probe around your chest to release soreness.

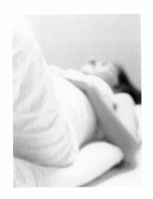

2 Stay lying down. With your feet flat on the floor and hip-width apart, push into your feet to lift your lower back off the ground. Support your hips with your hands for seven breaths and then take your arms overhead for another seven. Roll down slowly one vertebra at a time.

3 With feet flat on the floor, cross your right ankle over your left knee and let your legs drop to the right. Stretch your left arm over your head and look to your left hand. Repeat on the other side.

4 Lie on your left side with knees up and arms out in front of you. Take your right arm over to the opposite side, twisting your spine and taking your right shoulder closer to the floor. Hold for a few minutes, breathing into tense areas, and then repeat on the other side.

pamper your feet

As you read this, straighten and wiggle your toes. It's the quickest way to relieve tired, aching feet. At the end of a busy day, sit with your feet up for 10 minutes to improve circulation, or run yourself a foot bath (sit on the edge of your bath, or fill a bowl and get comfy on the couch). Soaking your feet in hot water containing two teaspoons of mustard will relieve aches and pains (and also helps treat a cold). Place a towel over your feet and ankles, and keep topping the hot water up to maintain the temperature for 15 minutes.

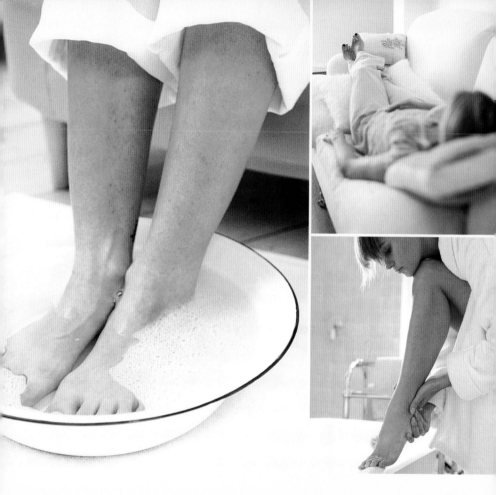

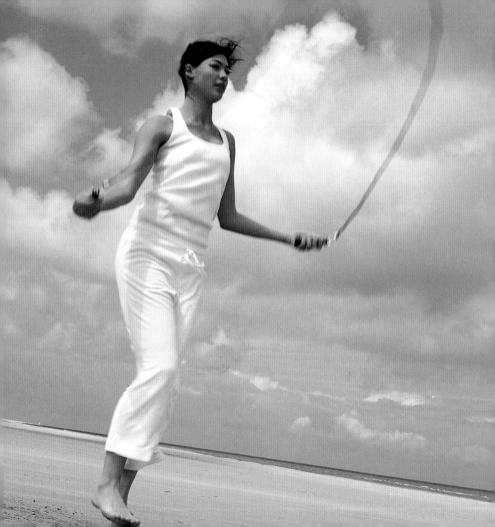

boost your mood

Background music has a huge effect on how we feel (as major retailers know only too well—everything they play is designed to get us buying). So get together a collection of soothing sounds (from mushy songs to Hari Krishna chanting—whatever works for you) and have them handy to restore your equilibrium after an overstimulated day. And, rather than a busy radio station or breakfast TV, start your day with something altogether calmer. You'll feel so much better for it.

Just 20 minutes of aerobic exercise will burn fat and release **HAPPY HORMONES** (research says stress symptoms can actually disappear within 20 minutes of starting a session). Don't have the time? A half-hour walk, five days a week, will use up only 2.2% of your total waking week. Alternatively, dance to loud music at home or power-walk with the stroller. You'll also be increasing your immunity—and losing weight without a single change to your diet.

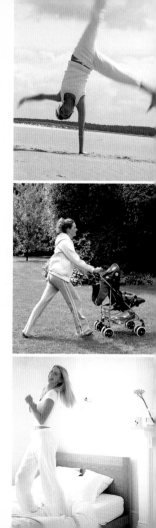

healing herbs

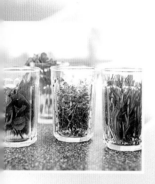

Ditch the drugs for minor complaints—herbs and spices are nature's natural healers. Add spices to your food and stock up on herbal teas (choose organic when possible). You can also make your own teas with herbs from the garden. Simply tear up a handful, put in a pot, cover with boiling water, and let brew for five minutes.

CAMOMILE, FENNEL, NETTLE, AND DANDELION TEAS Drink whenever you need to calm down and relax.

CAYENNE Warms up the circulation and also helps clear congested lungs.

CHILE Sweats out toxins when you want to detox or purge a cold.

GARLIC Nature's antibiotic, it works against colds and other infections and also helps lower blood pressure.

GINGER Warming and antiviral, use it fresh (or drink the tea) to relieve stomach problems including nausea, constipation, and indigestion.

PEPPERMINT Makes the perfect after-dinner drink, as it aids digestion and soothes a too-full stomach.

ROSEMARY Helps soothe a sore throat and sharpen a tired mind (inhale rosemary essential oil when you feel yourself flagging).

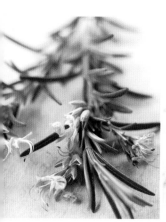
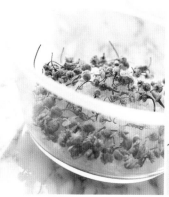
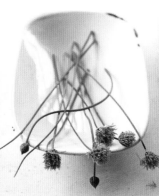

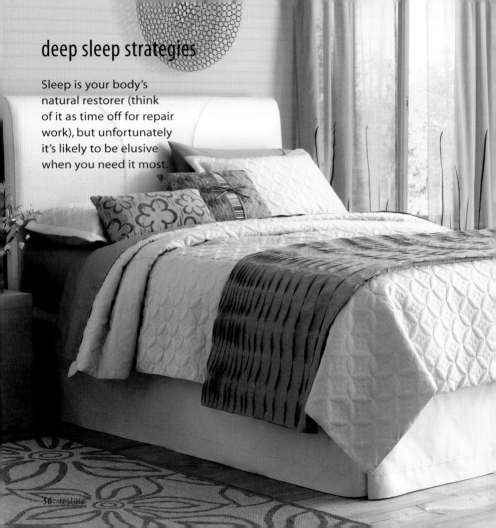

deep sleep strategies

Sleep is your body's natural restorer (think of it as time off for repair work), but unfortunately it's likely to be elusive when you need it most.

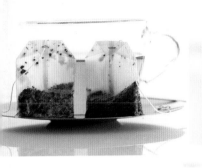

Drink a cup of soothing **CAMOMILE TEA** before bedtime or snack on a banana, which contains the sleep-inducing amino acid tryptophan. A **COLD FOOT BATH** will also help switch off your brain so you sleep more soundly. Immerse your feet and soak until the cold temperature becomes quite uncomfortable. Make the run-up to bedtime **RELAXING** (you can't expect to fall asleep 10 minutes after turning off a horror movie), and, if you still find yourself lying awake an hour later, stop trying to sleep. The worst thing you can do is concentrate on sleeping (you're still stimulating your brain), so recognize that falling asleep is out of your control and accept that lying there relaxing is the next best thing. That's about the time you'll drop off.

eat for energy

Essential fatty acids (EFAs) aren't called essential for nothing. Once you feel the impact omega 3 and 6 have on your stress levels, you'll never want to stop. Nearly a quarter of your brain's structure is composed of fatty acids, making them vital for brain health (from a good memory to fighting depression). They also boost immunity by giving your body energy to fend off harmful viruses and bacteria. And if you've ever suffered from dry skin or brittle nails, problem solved. We don't

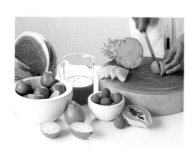

manufacture EFAs; you need to get them from food. Nuts, seeds, grains, legumes, vegetables, and fruit are good sources of omega 6; linseeds, pumpkin seeds, dark green vegetables, and cold-water oily fish such as salmon, sardines, mackerel, and tuna are good for omega 3. Tired all the time? You soon won't be.

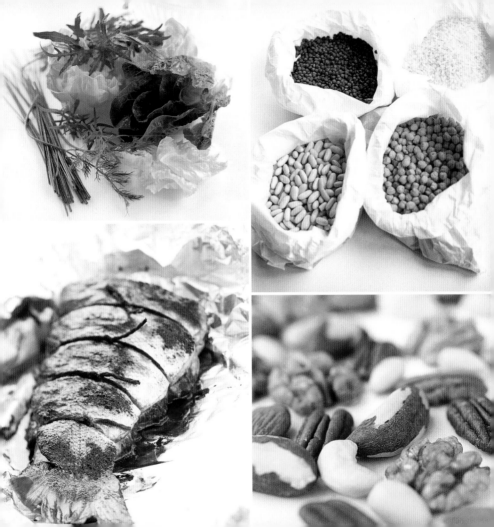

six ways to get your mojo back

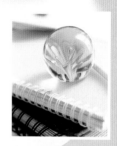

1 The way you think has a direct effect on how you look, so keep a notebook to record all the good things happening in your life: what other people say about you, and what you feel proud of doing yourself. Research says that positive thinking benefits every single cell in your body.

2 What excites you, both physically and emotionally? What do you love to do? What matters most to you? Making time for things you're enthusiastic about is very energizing.

3 No matter how many times you get knocked back, the secret of not remaining there is to try again. The more times you attempt to give up smoking or to exercise regularly, the more likely you'll do it. Be flexible and have a plan B. If you can't get to the gym three times a week, can you walk for 15 minutes every day?

4 Where have you let yourself down recently? By working too late? Drinking wine every night? Write down ways you can get back on course, and start keeping promises to yourself by making them small, manageable ones.

5 You have the same amount of energy you've always had, so if you constantly feel tired, chances are you're not using that energy wisely. Ask yourself: What am I doing that's adding to my energy reserves? What am I doing that's draining them? Now that you can see how you're creating your energy, how can you increase the day-to-day amount you have?

6 Before going to sleep, think of five things you're grateful for. Not only does gratitude feel good, it also contributes to an ongoing sense of happiness and wellbeing in your life.

credits

Key: ph=photographer, a=above, b=below, r=right, l=left, c=center

Endpapers ph David Montgomery; 1 ph Debi Treloar; 2–3 ph David Montgomery; 4 ph Alan Williams; 5 ph Polly Wreford; 7l & r ph David Montgomery; 7c ph Daniel Farmer; 8 ph David Montgomery; 9l ph Polly Wreford; 9r ph Henry Bourne; 10b & background ph David Montgomery; 10a & c ph Daniel Farmer; 11 ph David Montgomery; 12 ph Daniel Farmer; 13a ph Polly Wreford; 13b ph David Montgomery; 14 & 15a inset ph Dan Duchars; 15b inset ph Daniel Farmer; 15 background ph David Montgomery; 16 & 17a ph William Lingwood; 17b ph David Montgomery; 18 ph William Lingwood; 19–20 ph Dan Duchars; 21l ph David Montgomery; 21r–23l ph Daniel Farmer; 23c & r ph David Montgomery; 24–25 background ph David Montgomery; 24 inset ph Alan Williams; 25 inset ph James Merrell; 26l ph David Montgomery; 26r ph Chris Everard; 27al ph Peter Cassidy; 27ar ph Andrew Wood; 27b ph Christopher Drake; 28 ph David Montgomery; 29 ph Dan Duchars; 31al ph Noel Murphy; 31ac ph Jean Cazals; 31ar ph Nicki

Dowey; 31cr ph Peter Cassidy; 31bl ph Debi Treloar; 31bc ph Philip Webb; 31br

ph David Montgomery; 32–33 ph Claire Richardson; 34 background ph David

Montgomery; 34 inset & 35 ph Daniel Farmer; 36a ph Jan Baldwin; 36b ph Debi

Treloar; 37 ph Dan Duchars; 38 ph Jan Baldwin; 39a ph Francesca Yorke; 39b ph

Debi Treloar; 40 ph Daniel Farmer; 41–42 ph David Montgomery; 43 ph Polly

Wreford; 44–45 background ph David Montgomery; 45r ph Daniel Farmer; 46a

inset ph Debi Treloar; 46b inset & background ph David Montgomery; 47 ph

Chris Everard; 48 ph David Montgomery; 49 ph Debi Treloar; 50 ph Polly Wreford;

51l & ar ph Dan Duchars; 51br ph Daniel Farmer; 52–53a ph Chris Everard; 53c ph

Dan Duchars; 53b ph Polly Wreford; 54–55c ph David Montgomery; 55l & r ph

Peter Cassidy; 56 Courtesy of Pier 1 Imports®; 57 inset ph David Montgomery;

57 background ph Debi Treloar; 58–59al ph Peter Cassidy; 59ar ph Philip Webb;

59bl ph William Lingwood; 59br ph Francesca Yorke; 60 inset ph Polly Wreford;

60 background ph Jan Baldwin; 61 ph Chris Tubbs; 62–63 ph David Montgomery;

64 ph David Montgomery.

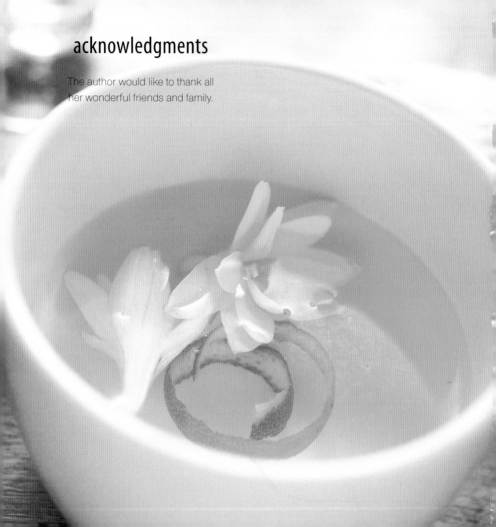

acknowledgments

The author would like to thank all
her wonderful friends and family.

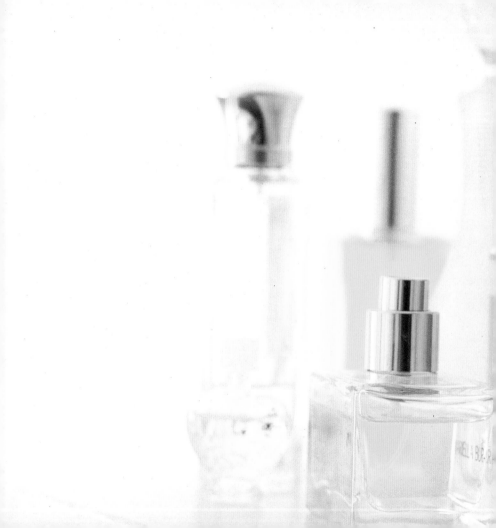